Chair Yoga for Seniors Over 60

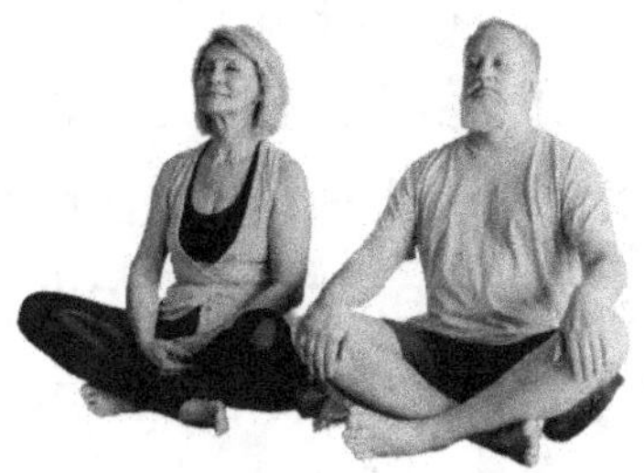

Revitalize Your Wellness from the comfort of a Seat

Jonathan M Sandra

DISCLAIMER

Acknowledgment

With immense gratitude, we extend our heartfelt appreciation to all those who contributed to the creation of this book. Our journey of bringing chair yoga for seniors to life has been a collaborative effort filled with inspiration, dedication, and shared passion for well-being.

We extend our deepest thanks to the seniors who have embraced this practice with open hearts, reminding us of the transformative power of mindful movement. Your stories and experiences have shaped the essence of this book.

To our editors and collaborators, your wisdom and guidance have enriched each page, ensuring that the information presented resonates authentically and meaningfully.

A special thank you to our families, friends, and loved ones for your unwavering support and encouragement throughout this endeavor.

Lastly, to the readers, we are honored to be a part of your wellness journey. May this book be a source of inspiration, comfort, and empowerment as you navigate the path of chair yoga and holistic well-being.

Dedication

To all the seniors who have embraced the journey of wellness with open hearts and curious minds. Your strength, resilience, and commitment to self-care have been an inspiration, showing us that age is just a number and that the path to well-being is an eternal one. This book is dedicated to each person who has taken a step on the path of chair yoga, seeking balance, mindfulness, and vitality.

May the pages of this book serve as a reminder of your inner strength and the beauty that comes from nurturing your body and mind. Your dedication to your well-being is a testament to the power of self-love and the boundless potential that resides within. As you explore the poses, breathe mindfully, and embrace the tranquility of each moment, may you continue to find joy, peace, and a deeper connection with yourself.

Table of Contents

Introduction

Welcome to the transformative world of "Chair Yoga for Seniors over 60: Revitalize Your Wellness from the Comfort of a Seat." Within these pages, you'll embark on a remarkable journey that defies the boundaries of age and invigorates your body, mind, and spirit.

Imagine a practice that rekindles your vitality, soothes your joints, and nurtures your inner calm, all while embracing the gentle embrace of a chair. Whether you're an experienced yogi or stepping into the realm of wellness for the first time, this guide is your compass to rediscovering the joys of movement, the serenity of breath, and the art of holistic living.

As the years gracefully unfold, our bodies may change, but our zest for life remains unwavering. "Chair Yoga for Seniors over 60" is not just a collection of poses; it's a celebration of the resilient spirit that defines each of us. We invite you to embrace this practice with open arms, honoring the unique journey that has brought you here.

In the pages ahead, you'll uncover an array of seated postures thoughtfully curated to rejuvenate your physical strength, restore balance, and ignite a renewed sense of purpose. Whether you're seeking relief from everyday stiffness or a moment of quiet introspection, each pose is a doorway to a more vibrant, flexible, and tranquil you.

But this guide is more than just movements; it's a roadmap to holistic well-being. You'll explore the art of mindful breathing, cultivating inner peace with each inhale and exhale. Through guided relaxation and meditation, you'll tap into reservoirs of serenity you never knew existed.

Join us as we navigate the enchanting landscapes of chair yoga, where age is but a number and possibilities are endless. Your chair becomes your sanctuary, your breath becomes your companion, and every movement becomes an ode to the joy of living fully.

So, dear reader, take a seat and immerse yourself in the chapters that follow. Let the wisdom of ancient practices and the embrace of your chair weave together a tapestry of well-lived moments. Let's embark on this voyage together where the only requirement is an open heart and the willingness to be transformed. Your journey to rejuvenation begins now.

Chapter 1

Benefits of chair Yoga for seniors

1. Age-Defying Flexibility: Chair yoga gracefully rekindles your body's flexibility, gently releasing tension and stiffness. Each pose encourages the freedom of movement, helping you maintain your youthful range of motion.

2. Revitalized Energy: Experience a surge of newfound vitality as chair yoga sequences stimulate blood flow and invigorate your muscles. Say goodbye to lethargy and hello to a more energized you.

3. Joint Nurturing: Discover a sanctuary for your joints as you seamlessly transition between poses. Chair yoga offers support, allowing you to enjoy the benefits of movement without added strain on your joints.

4. Peaceful Mind: Delve into moments of serene contemplation with mindful breathing and meditation. Experience tranquility as your mind unfurls its layers and finds solace in the stillness.

5. Stress Elixir: Chair yoga is your antidote to the hustle and bustle of life. Find release from daily stressors as you melt into poses, releasing tension and embracing a newfound sense of calm.

6. Balanced Body: Enhance your equilibrium and stability as chair yoga refines your balance and core strength. Feel confident and secure as you move through life's various terrains.

7. Mind-Body Connection: Immerse yourself in the exquisite harmony of mind and body. Each pose is an opportunity to reconnect with yourself, fostering a deeper appreciation for the present moment.

8. Heartfelt Health: Embrace the cardiovascular benefits of chair yoga, promoting heart health through gentle, rhythmic movements that help keep your circulation in check.

9. Digestive Harmony: Encourage healthy digestion with poses that massage your internal organs, supporting a well-functioning digestive system.

10. Social Connection: Chair yoga classes foster a sense of community, creating an environment where you can forge friendships, share stories, and find joy in the company of others on a similar journey.

11. Adaptable Wellness: Chair yoga celebrates your unique needs and abilities. Every pose can be tailored to suit your comfort, making this practice a versatile treasure for all.

12. Elevated Mood: Elevate your spirits and cultivate a positive outlook on life. Chair yoga's blend of movement and mindfulness can elevate your mood and leave you feeling uplifted.

13. Ageless Exploration: Chair yoga opens doors to exploration without boundaries. Whether you're a beginner or have practiced yoga for years, this practice offers a realm of new possibilities.

14. Empowerment: Celebrate your body's resilience and the empowerment that comes with nurturing your well-being. Chair yoga is a testament to your commitment to living life to its fullest.

Step into the world of chair yoga for seniors, where the chair becomes your partner in well-being, and each pose a testament to your enduring spirit. Let the captivating benefits transform not only your body but also your outlook on life itself.

Safety Precautions and Guidelines for Chair Yoga Practitioners:

1. Consult Your Healthcare Professional: Before starting any new exercise routine, including chair yoga, it's essential to consult your healthcare provider, especially if you have any pre-existing health conditions or concerns.

2. Listen to Your Body: Pay close attention to how your body feels during the practice. If you experience pain, discomfort, or dizziness, stop immediately and adjust the pose or take a break.

3. Stay within Your Comfort Zone: Chair yoga is about gentle movement and stretching. Never force yourself into a pose that feels uncomfortable or beyond your range of motion.

4. Use a Stable Chair: Choose a sturdy chair without wheels, and make sure it's placed on a flat, non-slip surface. Avoid using chairs with arms that are too wide or too narrow for your comfort.

5. Secure Clothing and Accessories: Wear comfortable clothing that allows you to move freely. Remove any loose jewelry or accessories that might get in the way during the practice.

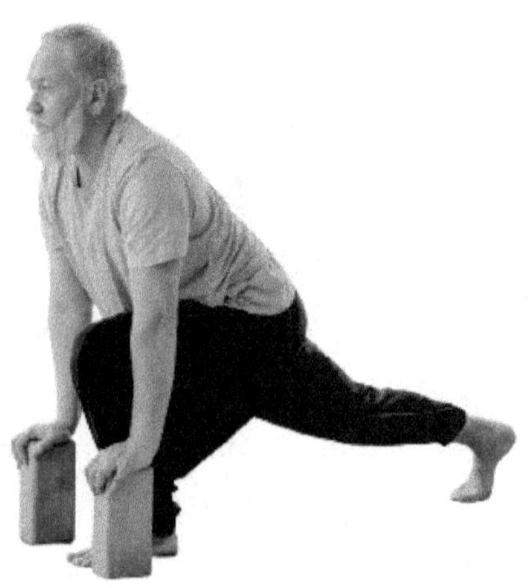

6. Proper Alignment: Focus on maintaining proper alignment in each pose. Align your body to prevent strain on joints and muscles.

7. Breath Awareness: Coordinate your breath with movement. Breathe naturally and avoid holding your breath. Breathing mindfully can help you relax and deepen your stretches.

8. Warm-Up Gradually: Start with gentle warm-up movements to prepare your body for more challenging poses. Gradually progress into deeper stretches as your body becomes more responsive.

9. Props for Support: Keep yoga props like cushions, blankets, or blocks nearby. These can provide extra support, especially if you have limited mobility.

10. Modifications Are Welcome: Your instructor might offer modifications for poses to suit your needs. Don't hesitate to use these modifications to ensure your safety and comfort.

11. Hydration: Stay hydrated before, during, and after your practice. Sip water as needed to keep your body refreshed.

12. Rest and Recovery: Incorporate rest periods between poses if necessary. Remember, it's okay to pause, take a breath, and reset before continuing.

13. Avoid Overexertion: While yoga encourages growth, avoid pushing yourself too hard, especially if you're just starting. Progress gradually to avoid strain or injury.

14. Regular Practice: Consistency is key. Engage in regular chair yoga sessions to experience the cumulative benefits. However, always respect your body's limitations.

15. Cool Down: End your practice with a gentle cool-down period to help your body relax and recover. Focus on deep, relaxed breathing during this time.

16. Mindful Exit: After your practice, stand up slowly if needed, and take a moment to notice how you feel. If you feel lightheaded, sit back down and take your time.

Remember, chair yoga is meant to enhance your well-being, not create stress or discomfort. By following these safety precautions and guidelines, you can enjoy the practice safely and derive the maximum benefit from it. If you're ever unsure about a pose or sensation, consult your instructor for guidance.

Choosing the Right Chair for Your Chair Yoga Practice:

Choosing the Right Chair for Your Chair Yoga Practice:

Selecting the appropriate chair for your chair yoga practice is essential to ensure comfort, stability, and safety. The chair becomes an integral part of your practice, supporting you as you explore gentle stretches and poses. Here's a guide to help you choose the right chair:

1. Sturdiness: Opt for a chair that is sturdy and stable. It should be able to support your weight without wobbling or tilting. Avoid chairs with wheels, as they may not provide the necessary stability.

2. Flat Seat: Look for a chair with a flat, even seat surface. This provides a comfortable base for your yoga poses. Chairs with padded seats can add an extra layer of comfort.

3. Armrests: Choose a chair with armrests that are at a comfortable height and width. Armrests can be used for

Chapter 2

Getting Started

Support in certain poses, so ensure they don't hinder your movement

4. Backrest Height: The backrest of the chair should be at a height that supports your spine without causing discomfort. It shouldn't be too low or too high, allowing you to sit with a neutral spine.

5. Seat Height: Ideally, the seat of the chair should be at a height where your feet can rest flat on the floor comfortably. This helps you maintain stability and balance during your practice.

6. Width and Depth: Consider the width and depth of the chair seat. You should have enough room to comfortably sit and move without feeling cramped.

7. No Sharp Edges: Ensure that the chair has no sharp edges or protruding parts that could cause discomfort or injury during your practice.

8. Material and Texture: The material of the chair's seat should be comfortable against your skin. Avoid chairs with slippery or rough surfaces that could lead to discomfort or instability.

9. No Reclining Feature: Chairs with a reclining feature might not provide the necessary support for chair yoga poses. Choose a chair that remains upright and stable.

10. Personal Preference: Ultimately, your comfort is paramount. Sit on the chair and assess how it feels to you. If it feels supportive, comfortable, and conducive to movement, it's likely a good choice.

11. Chair Legs: Check that the chair legs are even and in good condition. Uneven legs can cause the chair to wobble, affecting your stability.

12. Mobility: If you have limited mobility, look for a chair with arms that allow you to easily get in and out of the chair.

Remember that the chair you choose should enhance your practice, providing the necessary support and comfort for your movements. It's recommended to try out different chairs and find the one that best suits your body's needs. With the right chair as your ally, your chair yoga practice can be an enjoyable and beneficial experience.

Creating a Comfortable Environment for Your Chair Yoga Practice

Setting the stage for your chair yoga practice involves more than just finding the right chair. Crafting a comfortable environment contributes to a more enjoyable and fulfilling practice. Here's how to create a soothing atmosphere for your sessions:

1. Clothing Choice: Wear loose-fitting, comfortable clothing that allows you to move freely. Choose fabrics that are breathable and won't restrict your movement during poses.

2. Footwear: Practice chair yoga barefoot or with non-slip socks to maintain stability and traction on the floor.

3. Temperature Control: Ensure the room temperature is conducive to your comfort. Dress in layers so you can adjust as needed during your practice.

4. Noise Reduction: Find a quiet space where you can practice without distractions. If external noise is unavoidable, consider using soft instrumental music or white noise to mask disturbances.

5. Lighting: Opt for soft, natural lighting. Avoid harsh, direct lighting that could strain your eyes or create discomfort.

6. Ventilation: Adequate ventilation is essential to prevent overheating during your practice. Ensure fresh air circulates through the room.

7. Declutter: Clear the space around your chair of any unnecessary items. This helps prevent accidents and allows you to move without obstruction.

8. Personal Items: Keep a water bottle and a towel nearby in case you need them. Having these essentials within reach ensures you can stay hydrated and wipe away any sweat.

9. Props and Cushions: Have any yoga props or cushions you might need within arm's reach. These items can enhance your comfort and support in certain poses.

10. Aromatherapy: If you enjoy it, consider using calming scents through essential oils or candles. A calming environment can be created with fragrances like lavender or chamomile.

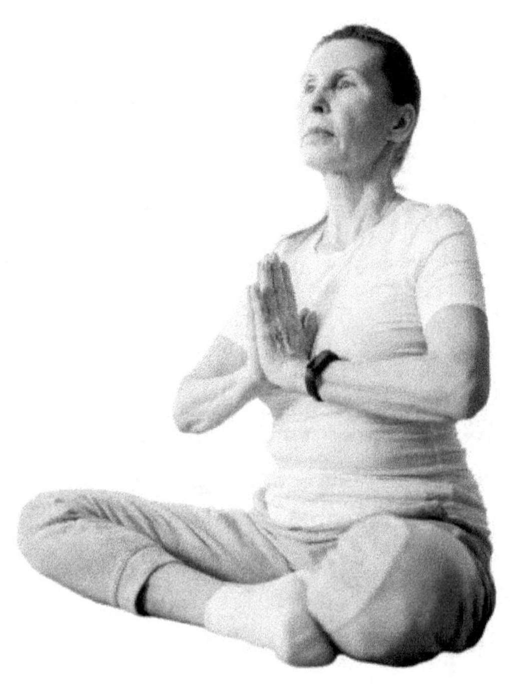

11. Technology: Turn off notifications on your devices to avoid interruptions. If you're following an online class, set up your device at a comfortable viewing angle.

12. Personalization: Decorate your practice area with items that bring you joy and tranquility, such as plants, artwork, or inspirational quotes.

13. Personal Space: Designate a specific spot for your chair yoga practice. Having a dedicated space helps signal to your mind that it's time for self-care.

14. Time Management: Set aside a consistent time for your chair yoga practice. This routine can help you make it a regular part of your day.

Creating a comfortable environment for chair yoga is about optimizing every aspect of your space to support your practice. By attending to these details, you'll be able to fully immerse yourself in the soothing embrace of your practice, finding peace, rejuvenation, and connection in every session.

Basic chair yoga poses

Here are some basic chair yoga poses that you can start with. Remember to focus on your breath, move gently, and only go as far as feels comfortable for your body.

1. Seated Mountain Pose:
  - Sit up straight in the chair, feet flat on the floor.
- Let your shoulders drop, then put your hands on your thighs.
  - Take a few deep breaths and close your eyes to feel anchored.

2. Seated Cat-Cow Stretch:
- Take a deep breath in and raise your chest (Cow).
   Exhale, arch your back, and tuck your chin into your chest (Cat).
  - Repeat these motions while breathing.

3. Seated Forward Fold:
- Exhale and stretch your spine.
   Exhale, lean forward at the hips, and tuck your legs over.

  - Let your head and arms hang loosely. Hold for a few breaths.

4. Seated Twist:
   - Sit up tall, place your left hand on your right knee.
   - Inhale, lengthen your spine.
   - Exhale, twist to the right, looking over your right shoulder.
   - Hold for a few breaths, then switch sides.

5. Seated Side Stretch:
   - Sit up straight, raise your left arm overhead.
   - Inhale, lengthen your spine.
   - Exhale, lean to the right, feeling a stretch along your left side.
   - Hold for a few breaths, then switch sides.

6. Ankle and Wrist Circles:
   - Lift your feet off the ground and circle your ankles in both directions.
   - Extend your arms and circle your wrists in both directions.

7. Seated Pigeon Pose:
   - - Position your left thigh over your right ankle.
8. Shoulder Opener:
- Place your hands together in a fist behind your back.
   - Inhale, lift your chest, and gently squeeze your shoulder blades together.
   - Hold for a few breaths.

9. Chair Warrior I:

- Your right foot should be placed forward as you sit on the chair's edge.

- Inhale, raise your arms overhead.
- Exhale, bend your right knee and sink into a lunge position.
- After a few breaths of holding, switch sides.

10. Chair Savasana (Relaxation):
- Sit comfortably with your back supported by the chair.
- Close your eyes, rest your hands on your lap, and take slow, deep breaths.
- Relax into the chair, releasing tension from head to toe.

These basic chair yoga poses are a wonderful starting point for your practice. As you become more comfortable, you can explore additional poses and sequences that suit your needs and abilities. Always remember to prioritize your safety and comfort while practicing.

Chapter 3

Breath Awareness and Relaxation

Gentle Breathing exercise

Gentle breathing exercise that you can practice to promote relaxation and mindfulness

4-7-8 Breathing:

1. Find a comfortable seated position in your chair, with your feet flat on the ground and your hands resting on your thighs.

2. Close your eyes and take a moment to settle into the present moment.

3. Inhale quietly through your nose for a count of 4 seconds. As you breathe in and out, you'll notice your stomach rising.

4. Hold your breath for a count of 7 seconds. During this pause, focus on the stillness and the sensation of holding your breath.

5. Exhale completely and audibly through your mouth for a count of 8 seconds. As you exhale, imagine releasing any tension or stress.

6. This completes one cycle of 4-7-8 breathing. Repeat this cycle for a few rounds, or as many times as you feel comfortable.

7. After your last cycle, take a few natural breaths and observe how you feel.

This breathing exercise can help activate the body's relaxation response, calming the nervous system and reducing stress. It's a simple practice that can be done anytime, anywhere, and is particularly helpful during moments of anxiety or when you need to unwind.

Progressive muscle relaxation

A relaxation technique called progressive muscle relaxation (PMR) includes gradually tensing and then relaxing various muscle groups in the body. It's a great way to release physical tension and promote relaxation. Here's how you can practice it:

1. Set the Scene: Find a quiet and comfortable place to sit or lie down. Wear loose and comfortable clothing.

2. Breathing: Take a few deep breaths to help you relax and focus your mind.

3. Progressive Muscle Relaxation Steps:

   a. Toes: Start with your toes. Curl them tightly for a few seconds, then release. As you let go, let the stress flow away.

   b. Feet: Point your toes away from you, feeling the stretch in your calf muscles. Hold, and then release.

   c. Legs: Tense your calf muscles by pressing your heels down and lifting your toes towards you. Hold, then release.

   d. Thighs: Tighten your thigh muscles by pressing your knees together. Hold, then release.

   e. Hips and Buttocks: Squeeze your buttocks together. Hold, then release.

f. Stomach: Tighten your abdominal muscles. Hold, then release.

g. Chest and Back: Take a deep breath and arch your back slightly, feeling your chest and back muscles engage. Exhale and release.

h. Shoulders: Shrug your shoulders up towards your ears. Hold, then release.

i. Arms and Hands: Clench your fists and flex your forearm muscles. Hold, then release.

j. Neck: Gently press your head back into the chair or the floor. Hold, then release.

k. Face: Scrunch up your face, wrinkling your forehead and squinting your eyes. Hold, then release.

4. Whole Body Relaxation: After going through each muscle group, take a few moments to let your entire body relax. Feel the warmth and relaxation flowing through you.

5. Deep Breathing: Take a few deep breaths and observe the sensation of relaxation in your body.

6. Open Your Eyes: When you're ready, slowly open your eyes and take a moment to become aware of your surroundings.

Progressive Muscle Relaxation can be a powerful tool to reduce stress and promote a sense of calm. Regular practice can help you become more attuned to your body and better manage physical tension.

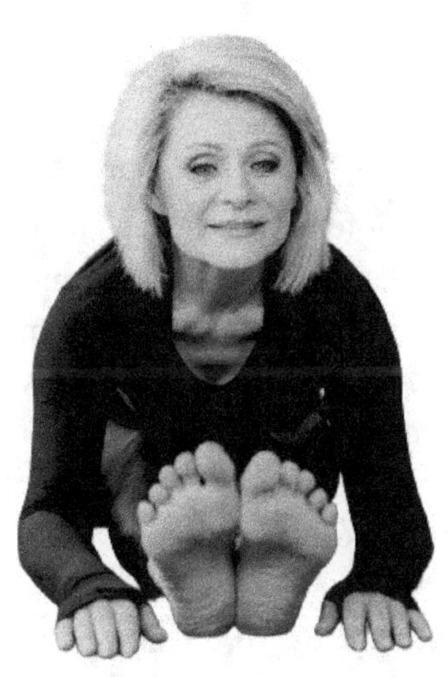

Chapter 4

Chair Yoga poses suitable for seniors

Seated Mountain Pose: Rediscovering Strength and Alignment

Seated Mountain Pose, a variation of the traditional Mountain Pose (Tadasana), is a foundational yoga pose that serves as the starting point for many seated chair yoga practices. Despite its seemingly simple appearance, this pose is a cornerstone for building strength, stability, and mindful awareness in your practice. Let's delve into the details of Seated Mountain Pose and its remarkable benefits.

Finding the Foundation:

1. Positioning: Begin by sitting comfortably in a sturdy chair with your feet flat on the ground and your spine erect. Your arms should rest comfortably on your thighs.

2. Alignment: Align your body so that your head, shoulders, and hips are in one vertical line.

3. Foot Placement: Place your feet hip-width apart and distribute your weight evenly between both feet. Feel a sense of grounding through your feet.

Unlocking the Benefits:

1. Postural Awareness: Seated Mountain Pose encourages you to be aware of your posture. It's an opportunity to realign your body, counteracting the effects of slouching or poor posture.

2. Spinal Health: The elongated spine in this pose helps maintain the natural curves of your spine, supporting good spinal health.

3. Stability: By sitting evenly on both sitting bones, you promote stability in your pelvis and encourage balanced weight distribution.

4. Core Activation: Engaging your core muscles while sitting tall helps improve core strength, essential for maintaining overall stability.

5. Breath Awareness: The simplicity of Seated Mountain Pose makes it an excellent platform for focusing on your breath. Mindful breathing promotes relaxation and helps you connect with the present moment.

6. Energizing: While seemingly static, this pose encourages a sense of upliftment. Visualize energy radiating through your body, promoting alertness and vitality.

Cultivating Mind-Body Connection

1. Intention: As you settle into Seated Mountain Pose, set an intention for your practice. It could be a sense of grounding, stability, or even just the intention to be present.

2. Mindfulness: This pose invites you to turn your attention inward. Notice the sensations in your body, the rhythm of your breath, and any areas of tension or relaxation.

3. Visual Imagery: Envision yourself as a mountain—strong, rooted, and unshakable. This imagery can enhance your sense of stability and resilience.

Adapting for Comfort

1. Cushions or Props: If needed, you can place a cushion under your sitting bones for added comfort or use a prop behind your lower back for support.

2. Arm Variation: Experiment with different arm positions. You can rest your hands on your thighs, place them on your lap, or try a palm-to-palm mudra for a more meditative touch.

Takeaways:

Seated Mountain Pose transcends its apparent simplicity, offering a myriad of benefits that extend far beyond the physical realm. It serves as a gateway to exploring mindfulness, postural awareness, and the innate strength within. Incorporate this pose into your chair yoga routine to lay the foundation for a practice that nurtures both body and mind.

Seated Cat-Cow Stretch: Nurturing Spinal Mobility and Relaxation

The Seated Cat-Cow Stretch, a variation of the classic Cat-Cow sequence, brings the essence of fluid movement and spinal articulation to your chair yoga practice. This gentle and accessible stretch provides a harmonious blend of flexibility, breath awareness, and relaxation. Let's delve into the nuances of the Seated Cat-Cow Stretch and how it can enhance your overall well-being.

Embracing the Essence:

1. Foundation: Begin in a seated position, comfortably resting on the edge of your chair. Place your feet hip-width apart, grounding them firmly on the floor.

2. Alignment: Align your spine in a neutral position, maintaining the natural curves of your lower back (lumbar), middle back (thoracic), and upper back (cervical).

3. Hand Placement: Rest your hands gently on your thighs, palms facing downward, ensuring a relaxed and neutral shoulder position.

The Cat-Cow Dance

1. Seated Cow (Inhale):
   - Inhale deeply and gradually arch your spine, lifting your chest and bringing your shoulder blades together.
   - Gently tilt your pelvis forward, creating a slight anterior pelvic tilt.
   - Let your head and tailbone lift slightly as your gaze turns upward.

2. Seated Cat (Exhale):
   - As you exhale, round your spine gently, starting from your tailbone and moving through each vertebra.
   - Drop your head toward your chest, allowing your chin to move closer to your collarbone.
   - Engage your core muscles slightly to support the rounding of your spine.

Benefits Beyond Flexibility

1. Spinal Mobility: The Seated Cat-Cow Stretch encourages the fluid movement of your spine, promoting flexibility and range of motion. This is particularly beneficial for seniors to counteract stiffness and maintain a supple spine.

2. Breath and Movement Fusion: Pairing breath with movement amplifies the benefits. The inhale during Seated Cow extends and opens the chest, while the exhale during Seated Cat facilitates relaxation and gentle compression of the spine.

3. Stress Reduction: The rhythmic flow of this stretch calms the nervous system, making it an effective tool for stress reduction and relaxation.

4. Postural Awareness: Practicing Seated Cat-Cow Stretch cultivates awareness of your spinal alignment and can counteract the effects of poor posture.

Integrating Mindfulness

1. Breath Sync: Pay attention to the synchronization of breath and movement. Inhale as you transition to Seated Cow and exhale as you move into Seated Cat.

2. Mind-Body Connection: While performing the stretch, direct your focus to the sensations in your spine. Notice the gentle expansion during Seated Cow and the soothing release during Seated Cat.

Adapting for Comfort:

1. Gentle Movements: Seniors can embrace a slower pace to honor their bodies and ensure comfort during the stretch.

2. Chair Support: If needed, you can place a cushion behind your lower back for added support.

Concluding Thoughts

The Seated Cat-Cow Stretch embodies the essence of fluidity and relaxation in a chair yoga practice. As you seamlessly transition between Seated Cow and Seated Cat, you'll discover a renewed sense of spinal vitality and a deeper connection between breath and movement. Incorporate this stretch into your routine to invigorate your body and cultivate a sense of tranquility.

Seated Forward Fold: Embrace Tranquility and Release Tension

The Seated Forward Fold, a cherished pose in both traditional yoga and chair yoga practices, offers a serene journey inward, a space for introspection, and a gentle invitation to unwind. This seated variation of the Forward Fold provides an opportunity for seniors to experience the benefits of this classic pose in a comfortable and supported manner. Let's delve into the world of the Seated Forward Fold and explore its numerous physical and mental advantages.

The Gateway to Stillness:

1. Foundation: Begin by sitting near the edge of your chair, with your feet flat on the ground and hip-width apart. Sit up tall, establishing a strong connection with the chair and the earth beneath you.

2. Alignment: Ensure your spine is erect and your shoulders are relaxed. Maintain a sense of length through your spine from the tailbone to the crown of your head.

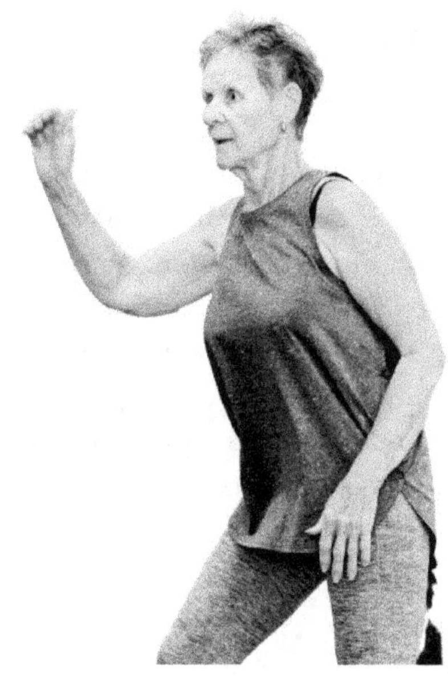

The journey of the Pose

1. Inhale: As you inhale deeply, lengthen your spine even more. Feel the gentle lift through the crown of your head.

2. Exhale: On your exhale, slowly hinge at your hips, leading with your chest, and fold forward over your legs. Allow your head and arms to drape down toward the floor.

3. Hands Placement: You can rest your hands on your thighs, shins, ankles, or even hold onto your feet. Find a position that allows you to relax into the stretch without strain.

4. Relaxation: In the folded position, take a moment to soften into the pose. Let go of any tension in your neck, shoulders, and spine. Stay in the position for a few breaths while taking deep breaths.

Physical and Emotional Release:

1. Hamstring Stretch: The Seated Forward Fold offers a gentle stretch to the hamstrings, promoting flexibility and mobility in the back of your legs.

2. Spinal Release: The forward folding action provides a subtle spinal decompression, releasing tension and creating space between the vertebrae.

3. Calm Mind: This pose encourages a calm and introspective state of mind. As you fold forward, you turn your gaze inward, nurturing a sense of quiet and tranquility.

4. Stress Reduction: The act of folding forward has a soothing effect on the nervous system, making it a valuable tool for stress reduction.

Mindful Exploration:

1. Breath Awareness: Pay attention to your breath as you fold forward. Inhale to create space, and exhale to relax deeper into the stretch.

2. Body Scan: Use this pose as an opportunity to scan your body for areas of tension. With each exhale, imagine releasing and letting go.

Adaptations for Comfort:

1. Chair Support: If reaching your feet feels challenging, use a strap or belt to loop around your feet, allowing you to gently pull yourself into the stretch.

2. Knee Comfort: If you have sensitive knees, consider placing a cushion or folded blanket under your knees for support.

Closing Thoughts:

The Seated Forward Fold is a gateway to stillness, a gesture of self-care that extends beyond the physical realm. As you gracefully fold forward, you create space for physical release and inner reflection. Infuse this pose into your chair yoga practice to nurture both your body and your spirit, fostering a sense of serenity and renewal.

Ankle Circles: A Gentle Revival for Mobility and Comfort

Ankle circles, a simple yet effective exercise, bring a delightful twist of movement to your chair yoga practice. These graceful rotations of the ankle joints offer a gentle way to improve flexibility, increase circulation, and alleviate discomfort. Let's embark on a journey into the world of ankle circles, discovering their benefits and embracing the freedom of fluid motion.

The Dance of Ankle Circles:

1. Initial Position: Begin by sitting comfortably in your chair with your feet flat on the ground, hip-width apart.

2. Foot Awareness: Direct your attention to your feet. Feel the connection between your soles and the earth beneath you.

3. Circling Motion: Slowly lift one foot off the ground, keeping your toes relaxed. Begin to trace a circle with your toes in a clockwise direction.

4. Explore the Range: As you circle, let your ankle joints move through their full range of motion. Gradually make the circles larger or smaller, finding the rhythm that feels most comfortable.

5. Switch Direction: After a few rotations, switch to counterclockwise circles, exploring the opposite direction.

6. Complete Set: Perform ankle circles on one foot for a few rounds, then gently place your foot back on the ground. On the opposite foot, repeat the sequence.

Benefits Beyond the Feet:

1. Ankle Mobility: Ankle circles promote the flexibility and mobility of the ankle joints, essential for walking, balance, and overall lower-body movement.

2. Circulation Enhancement: The gentle movement stimulates blood flow to the feet and lower legs, aiding in circulation and reducing the risk of swelling.

3. Joint Lubrication: By moving the ankle joints through their full range, you help distribute synovial fluid, which lubricates the joints and supports their health.

4. Alleviating Discomfort: Ankle circles can ease discomfort caused by prolonged sitting or conditions such as arthritis, offering a gentle way to relieve stiffness.

Mindful Movement:

1. Breath Connection: Coordinate your breath with the movement. Inhale as you lift your foot, and exhale as you circle.

2. Sensory Exploration: Pay attention to the sensations in your ankles as you perform the circles. Notice any areas of tension or areas that feel particularly free.

Incorporating Ankle Circles:

1. Chair Yoga Warm-Up: Begin your chair yoga session with ankle circles to awaken your feet and lower legs.

2. Midday Refresh: Incorporate ankle circles as a midday break to invigorate your circulation and provide a moment of mindful movement.

Adapting for Comfort:

1. Chair Support: If you have limited mobility, you can perform ankle circles while seated on the edge of your chair, using the chair for support.

2. Mindful Pace: Seniors can perform ankle circles at a pace that feels comfortable, ensuring a gentle and enjoyable experience.

Closing Thoughts:

Ankle circles are a testament to the beauty of simplicity in movement. Through this graceful dance of the ankles, you honor the well-being of your lower extremities and infuse your practice with a touch of mindful motion. Whether as part of your warm-up routine or a standalone exercise, ankle circles offer a reminder that even the smallest gestures can bring a profound sense of revitalization and comfort.

Wrist Circles: Nurturing Flexibility and Ease in Your Wrists

Wrist circles, like a soothing melody for your wrists, introduce a gentle and graceful movement to your chair yoga practice. These circular motions provide a refreshing way to enhance flexibility, increase blood flow, and alleviate tension in the wrists. Let's embark on a journey to discover the benefits and mindfulness of wrist circles, inviting a harmonious blend of motion and relaxation into your practice.

The Art of Wrist Circles:

1. Starting Position: Begin by sitting comfortably in your chair, with your spine erect and your feet grounded. Your hands should be on your thighs with the palms facing down.

2. Wrist Awareness: Direct your attention to your wrists. Feel the connection between your hands and your wrists, noticing any sensations present.

3. Creating Circles: Slowly lift one hand off your thigh and extend your arm forward, keeping your fingers relaxed. Begin to trace a gentle circle with your fingertips in a clockwise direction.

4. Exploring Movement: As you draw the circle, allow your wrist to move through its natural range of motion. You can make the circles larger or smaller, adapting to what feels comfortable for you.

5. Switching Direction: After a few rotations, reverse the direction, moving your fingertips counterclockwise to complete the circle.

6. Completing the Sequence: Perform wrist circles on one hand for a few rounds, then gently place your hand back on your thigh. Conversely, repeat the procedure.

Benefits Beyond the Wrists:

1. Wrist Flexibility: Wrist circles encourage flexibility in the wrist joints, vital for everyday activities that involve hand movement.

2. Blood Flow Enhancement: The circular motion stimulates blood circulation in the wrists and hands, supporting nourishment and oxygen delivery to the tissues.

3. Tension Release: Wrist circles can help alleviate tension and discomfort caused by prolonged typing, writing, or other activities that strain the wrists.

4. Joint Health: The gentle movement lubricates the wrist joints, promoting their health and reducing the risk of stiffness.

Mindful Flow:

1. Breath Awareness: Sync your breath with the movement. Inhale as you lift your hand, and exhale as you complete the circle.

2. Sensory Exploration: As you perform wrist circles, notice the sensations in your wrists. Pay attention to any areas of tightness or freedom of movement.

Integration in Your Practice

1. Warm-Up: Begin your chair yoga practice with wrist circles to awaken and prepare your wrists for movement.

2. Midday Break: Incorporate wrist circles as a quick and rejuvenating break from work or other activities.

Comfort and Adaptations:

1. Chair Support: If you have limited mobility, perform wrist circles while sitting at the edge of your chair, using the chair for support.

2. Gentle Pace: Seniors can perform wrist circles at a pace that feels comfortable, focusing on gentle and mindful movement.

Closing Reflection:

Wrist circles bring a soft and rhythmic touch to your practice, honoring the intricate workings of your wrists. Through these graceful circles, you offer your wrists a moment of care and attention, celebrating their mobility and vitality. Whether as a brief interlude in your day or a thoughtful addition to your chair yoga routine, wrist circles remind you of the beauty that lies in embracing movement with mindfulness and grace.

Seated Pigeon Pose: Nurturing Hip Flexibility and Comfort

Seated Pigeon Pose, a variation of the traditional Pigeon Pose, extends an invitation to gently open and release tension in the hips while honoring the comfort of a seated position. This pose offers seniors a way to enhance hip mobility, alleviate tightness, and foster a sense of ease. Let's explore the intricacies of Seated Pigeon Pose and the nurturing benefits it brings to your chair yoga practice.

Setting the Foundation:

1. Initial Position: Begin seated on the edge of your chair, both feet flat on the ground, and your spine tall and aligned.

2. Ankle Crossing: Lift your right ankle and place it over your left thigh, just above the knee. To safeguard your knee joint, bend your right foot.

3. Spinal Alignment: Ensure your spine remains straight and upright, maintaining the natural curves of your lower back.

Exploring the Pose

1. Gentle Lean: While keeping your back straight, gently lean forward from your hips. The goal is not to reach your toes but to feel a comfortable stretch in your right hip.

2. Hands Placement: You can rest your hands on your thighs, on the floor beside your chair, or on your raised foot for support.

3. Mindful Breath: Take slow and deep breaths, allowing the breath to guide you deeper into the stretch with each exhale.

4. Switch Sides: Release the right ankle from the left thigh, and repeat the sequence with the left ankle over the right thigh.

Benefits Beyond Flexibility

1. Hip Flexibility: Seated Pigeon Pose provides a gentle stretch to the hips, promoting flexibility and mobility in the hip joints.

2. Tension Release: This pose can help release tension in the hips and lower back, areas often affected by prolonged sitting.

3. Energetic Flow: Opening the hips can create an energetic flow, providing a sense of liberation and release.

4. Mindful Connection: As you direct your awareness to the sensations in your hips, you cultivate mindfulness and presence.

Mind-Body Integration

1. Breath Awareness: Inhale deeply as you prepare to lean forward, and exhale as you find a comfortable stretch in your hip.

2. Sensory Exploration: Tune into the sensations as you lean forward. Notice any areas of tightness or areas that respond well to the stretch.

Making It Yours:

1. Chair Support: If you have limited flexibility, use a cushion or prop under the raised knee for support.

2. Comfort Focus: The goal of Seated Pigeon Pose is to find a gentle stretch, not to force your body into a deep fold.

Reflection and Integration:

Seated Pigeon Pose is a reminder of the transformative power of gentle movements. Through this pose, you create a sacred space to nurture your hips and offer them a sense of liberation. Whether you practice it as a stand-alone stretch or as part of a comprehensive chair yoga routine, Seated Pigeon Pose is an invitation to honor your body's wisdom and explore the harmony of flexibility and comfort.

Shoulder Opener: Embrace Freedom and Release in Your Shoulders

The Shoulder Opener, a graceful and liberating movement, introduces a sense of spaciousness and ease into your chair yoga practice. This gentle stretch invites you to release tension, promote flexibility, and cultivate a sense of openness in your shoulder joints. Let's explore the beauty of the Shoulder Opener and the profound benefits it brings to your overall well-being.

Laying the Foundation:

1. Initial Position: Sit comfortably on the edge of your chair, with your spine tall and your feet grounded.

2. Hand Placement: Extend your arms forward at shoulder height, parallel to the ground. Put your palms together and spread your fingers widely.

3. Alignment: Keep your shoulders relaxed and your chest open, creating a broad and welcoming space in your upper body.

Exploring the Stretch

1. Inhale and Lift: As you inhale deeply, raise your arms to shoulder height, engaging your core muscles for stability.

2. Clasp Your Hands: Reach your arms wide, then clasp your hands behind your back, interlacing your fingers. If clasping isn't possible, hold onto a strap or the edge of your chair.

3. Shoulder Blades Together: Gently squeeze your shoulder blades together, feeling a stretch across your chest and the front of your shoulders.

4. Lift Your Chest: As you press your hands down and lift your chest, imagine a string gently pulling the crown of your head upward.

Benefits Beyond Flexibility:

1. Shoulder Mobility: The Shoulder Opener promotes mobility in the shoulder joints, reducing stiffness and enhancing overall shoulder function.

2. Chest Expansion: By opening the chest, you encourage better posture and create space for deeper breathing.

3. Stress Relief: The act of stretching and releasing tension in the shoulders can have a calming and stress-relieving effect.

4. Energetic Flow: Shoulder openers can create an energetic flow, helping to dissipate stagnant energy in the upper body.

Mindful Integration:

1. Breath Awareness: Inhale as you lift your arms and clasp your hands, and exhale as you gently press your hands down and lift your chest.

2. Sensory Exploration: As you hold the pose, notice the sensations in your shoulders and chest. Are there areas of tightness or areas that respond well to the stretch?

Adapting for Comfort:

1. Shoulder Sensitivity: If you have shoulder sensitivity or limited mobility, you can perform the stretch with your arms slightly lower or by gently holding onto the sides of your chair.

2. Gentle Pressure: Apply gentle pressure with your clasped hands, finding a level of stretch that feels comfortable and not overly intense.

Reflect and Integrate:

The Shoulder Opener is a gift you offer to your upper body an opportunity to unravel knots of tension, invite in freedom, and embrace the soothing embrace of release. Through this pose, you acknowledge the intricate balance between strength and surrender, cultivating a sense of harmony that echoes throughout your practice and your life. Incorporate the Shoulder Opener into your chair yoga routine, and let its gentle grace inspire a deeper connection with your body's wisdom and the beauty of mindful movement.

Seated Warrior I: Cultivating Strength and Grounding in Your Practice

Seated Warrior I, a modified version of the traditional Warrior I pose, brings a touch of empowerment and stability to your chair yoga practice. This seated variation offers seniors a way to build strength, enhance focus, and connect with a sense of groundedness. Let's delve into the essence of Seated Warrior I and discover the enriching benefits it brings to your practice.

Establishing the Foundation:

1. Initial Position: Begin by sitting near the edge of your chair, with your spine tall and your feet firmly grounded.

2. Leg Position: Extend your right leg forward, with your foot flexed and toes pointing toward the ceiling.

3. Bent Knee: Bend your left knee and place your left foot on the ground, positioning it outside the edge of your chair.

Exploring the Pose:

1. Engage Your Core: Draw your navel gently toward your spine to engage your core muscles.

2. Inhale and Raise: As you inhale deeply, raise your arms overhead, reaching toward the sky. Keep your shoulders relaxed.

3. Exhale and Lean: On your exhale, gently lean your upper body toward your right leg. Avoid collapsing the chest; instead, maintain an open chest and a long spine.

4. Grounding: Feel the connection between your seated hip and the grounded foot. Imagine yourself rooted and steady, like a warrior grounded in their strength.

Benefits Beyond Strength:

1. Strength Building: Seated Warrior I engages the muscles of your legs, core, and arms, promoting strength and stability.

2. Energizing: The act of raising your arms and opening your chest can have an invigorating and energizing effect.

3. Grounding and Focus: This pose encourages a sense of grounded focus, helping you connect with your inner strength and presence.

4. Posture Enhancement: By practicing Seated Warrior I, you promote good posture and alignment in your upper body.

Mindful Embodiment:

1. Breath Connection: Inhale as you raise your arms, and exhale as you lean toward your leg.

2. Sensory Awareness: As you lean into the stretch, notice the sensations in your hips, the stretch along your sides, and the grounding of your foot.

Comfort and Adaptations:

1. Chair Support: If you have limited mobility or balance concerns, perform the pose with your foot on the ground and your hands resting on your thigh.

2. Gentle Incline: Instead of leaning too far forward, focus on a gentle and comfortable incline to protect your lower back.

Integration and Reflection:

Seated Warrior I invites you to embody the strength and resilience of a warrior while respecting the uniqueness of your own body. Through this pose, you embrace both your physical strength and your inner fortitude, creating a harmonious blend of power and grace. Integrate Seated Warrior I into your chair yoga practice, allowing its essence to infuse your movements with intention and reminding you that within every pose, you have the opportunity to cultivate a deeper connection with yourself.

Seated Warrior II: Embodying Balance and Expansion

Seated Warrior II, a modified rendition of the classic Warrior II pose, brings a sense of equilibrium and expansive energy to your chair yoga practice. This seated variation offers seniors a way to cultivate balance, enhance focus, and experience the sensation of opening up to the world around them. Let's delve into the essence of Seated Warrior II and uncover the enriching benefits it brings to your practice.

Creating the Foundation:

1. Initial Position: Begin by sitting comfortably near the edge of your chair, with your spine erect and your feet grounded.

2. Leg Position: Extend your right leg forward, with your foot flexed and toes pointing toward the ceiling.

3. Bent Knee: Bend your left knee and place your left foot on the ground, positioning it outside the edge of your chair.

Exploring the Pose:

1. Engage Your Core: Gently activate your core muscles by drawing your navel in toward your spine.

2. Arms Position: Extend your arms out to the sides at shoulder height, parallel to the ground. Your palms should face down.

3. Gaze Direction: Direct your gaze over your left fingertips, allowing your gaze to rest gently on the horizon.

4. Open Your Hips: As you open your hips to the left, find a comfortable position that allows your left knee to align with your left ankle.

Benefits Beyond Balance:

1. Balance Cultivation: Seated Warrior II encourages balance and stability as you ground your left foot and extend your arms.

2. Focus Enhancement: The directed gaze promotes focus and presence, helping you cultivate a centered state of mind.

3. Side Body Stretch: The extended arms and open chest create a gentle stretch along the sides of your body.

4. Inner Expansion: Seated Warrior II invites you to expand your awareness outward, as if embracing the vastness of the world around you.

Mindful Presence:

1. Breath Alignment: Inhale deeply as you extend your arms, and exhale as you ground your foot and settle into the pose.

2. Sensory Connection: Notice the sensations in your hips, your extended arms, and the gentle stretch along your side body.

Comfort and Adaptations:

1. Chair Support: If you prefer more support or have limited mobility, practice the pose with your hands on your thighs and focus on the open chest and hip alignment.

2. Gentle Stretch: While seated, focus on the sensation of expansion in your arms and side body without straining.

Integration and Reflection:

Seated Warrior II encourages you to embrace balance and expansion from the comfort of your chair. Through this pose, you embody the qualities of a warrior—steadiness, awareness, and the ability to open your heart to the world. Incorporate Seated Warrior II into your chair yoga practice, allowing its essence to permeate your movements and infuse your practice with a sense of empowerment and grace. As you expand your arms and your awareness, remember that within every pose lies an opportunity to cultivate both inner and outer harmony.

Seated Tree Pose: Nurturing Balance and Connection

Seated Tree Pose, a modified adaptation of the traditional Tree Pose, invites you to find balance and connection while rooted in your chair. This seated variation offers seniors a way to explore stability, cultivate mindfulness, and feel the grounding essence of a tree. Let's delve into the essence of Seated Tree Pose and uncover the enriching benefits it brings to your chair yoga practice.

Establishing a Rooted Foundation:

1. Initial Position: Sit comfortably on the edge of your chair, with your spine elongated and your feet grounded.

2. Grounding: Feel the connection between your feet and the floor, drawing energy downward as if you were growing roots.

Exploring the Pose:

1. Engage Your Core: Gently engage your core muscles to support your posture and balance.

2. Foot Placement: Place your right foot on your left inner thigh, above the knee. If this is challenging, you can place your right foot on your left ankle or calf.

3. Hands Position: Rest your hands on your lap, allowing them to rest in a comfortable and relaxed position.

4. Balancing Act: Find a focal point in front of you to gaze at, helping you maintain balance and focus.

5. Lengthen Your Spine: Imagine a string pulling you gently upward from the crown of your head, lengthening your spine.

Benefits Beyond Balance:

1. Balance Cultivation: Seated Tree Pose encourages balance and stability while sitting, fostering a sense of grounding and centeredness.

2. Mindful Presence: The act of finding balance requires focused attention, helping you cultivate mindfulness.

3. Connection to Nature: The imagery of a tree encourages you to connect with the rooted stability of nature, even while sitting indoors.

4. Leg Awareness: You'll become more aware of the alignment and sensations in your legs as you balance.

Mindful Embodiment:

1. Breath Awareness: Inhale deeply as you prepare to lift your foot, and exhale as you find your balance.

2. Sensory Connection: Feel the gentle pressure of your foot against your thigh and notice any adjustments you make to maintain your balance.

Comfort and Adaptations:

1. Chair Support: If lifting your leg feels challenging, you can rest your right foot on your left calf or ankle for a more accessible variation.

2. Hand Position: If needed, hold onto the sides of the chair for added support while practicing Seated Tree Pose.

Integration and Reflection:

Seated Tree Pose is a reminder that the essence of a pose can be felt in even the simplest of movements. Through this pose, you tap into the stability and beauty of a tree's presence, embracing both your own inner strength and your connection to the world around you. Integrate Seated Tree Pose into your chair yoga practice, allowing it to infuse your movements with intention and serve as a gentle reminder that, like a tree, you too can find balance and rootedness within every moment.

Seated Bridge Pose: Fostering Spinal Mobility and Comfort

Seated Bridge Pose, a variation of the classic Bridge Pose, brings a sense of gentle openness and relaxation to your chair yoga practice. This seated adaptation offers seniors a way to create space in the spine, alleviate tension, and promote a comfortable sense of release. Let's explore the essence of Seated Bridge Pose and uncover the soothing benefits it brings to your practice.

Setting the Foundation:

1. Initial Position: Begin by sitting comfortably on the edge of your chair, with your feet flat on the ground and your spine tall.

2. Hand Placement: Place your hands on the sides of your chair, near your hips, with your fingers pointing forward.

Exploring the Pose:

1. Engage Your Core: Gently engage your core muscles by drawing your navel in toward your spine.

2. Press and Lift: As you inhale, press into your hands and feet. Lift your hips slightly off the chair, creating a gentle arch in your lower back.

3. Gentle Extension: Allow your head to drop back slightly if it's comfortable, without straining your neck.

4. Maintain Comfort: Find a height for your bridge that feels comfortable and accessible, without overextending your spine.

Benefits Beyond Release:

1. Spinal Release: Seated Bridge Pose encourages gentle extension of the spine, promoting a sense of openness and mobility.

2. Shoulder and Hip Flexibility: As you press into your hands, you can experience a gentle stretch in the shoulders. The pose also engages the hip flexors.

3. Stress Relief: The supported arch of the back can have a soothing effect on the nervous system, making it a valuable relaxation tool.

4. Chest Opening: Seated Bridge Pose creates space across the chest, encouraging better posture and improved breathing.

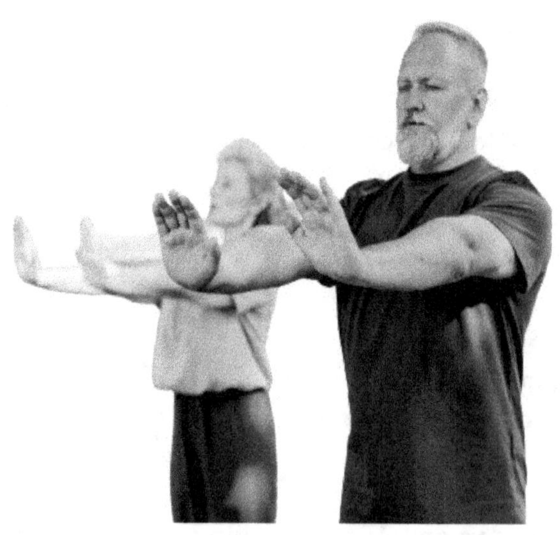

Mindful Connection

1. Breath Alignment: Inhale as you press into your hands and feet, and exhale as you release the pose and lower your hips.

2. Sensory Awareness: As you lift your hips, notice the sensation in your lower back, hips, and shoulders. Pay attention to any adjustments you make to find comfort.

Comfort and Adaptations:

1. Chair Support: If you have mobility concerns, you can practice a gentler version by lifting your hips only slightly off the chair.

2. Head Position: If dropping your head back feels uncomfortable, maintain a neutral head position or look forward.

Integration and Reflection:

Seated Bridge Pose is a reminder that even while sitting, you can create space and a sense of release in your body. Through this pose, you honor the natural curves of your spine and offer yourself a gentle stretch and relaxation. Infuse Seated Bridge Pose into your chair yoga practice, allowing it to be a gentle gateway to spinal mobility, a connection to your breath, and an invitation to find comfort and ease within the embrace of your practice.

Seated Butterfly Stretch: Embracing Flexibility and Ease

The Seated Butterfly Stretch, a variation of the classic Butterfly Pose, invites you to open your hips and release tension while comfortably seated in your chair. This gentle stretch offers seniors a way to enhance hip flexibility, promote relaxation, and experience the sensation of unfolding like a butterfly's wings. Let's explore the essence of the Seated Butterfly Stretch and uncover the nurturing benefits it brings to your chair yoga practice.

Creating a Gentle Foundation:

1. Initial Position: Sit comfortably on the edge of your chair, with your spine elongated and your feet grounded.

2. Knee Placement: Bend both knees, allowing your feet to come together and the soles of your feet to touch.

3. Hand Placement: Place your hands on your thighs, with your palms facing down.

Exploring the Pose:

1. Engage Your Core: Gently engage your core muscles to support your posture and alignment.

2. Knee Movement: Allow your knees to gently drop toward the sides, opening your hips and creating a diamond shape with your legs.

3. Gentle Lean: If comfortable, lean forward slightly from your hips to enhance the stretch in your hips and inner thighs.

4. Maintain Comfort: Find a depth of stretch that feels comfortable and soothing, avoiding any sensations of strain.

Benefits Beyond Flexibility:

1. Hip Flexibility: Seated Butterfly Stretch encourages gentle opening of the hips, promoting flexibility and mobility.

2. Inner Thigh Release: The pose offers a soft stretch to the inner thighs, helping to alleviate tension caused by sitting for extended periods.

3. Relaxation: As you settle into the stretch, you create a sense of relaxation and tranquility, which can be soothing for both the body and mind.

4. Mind-Body Connection: Seated Butterfly Stretch invites you to listen to your body's cues and find the balance between effort and ease.

Mindful Unfolding:

1. Breath Awareness: Inhale deeply as you find your initial position, and exhale as you allow your knees to gently drop outward.

2. Sensory Exploration: As you lean forward, notice the sensations in your hips, inner thighs, and lower back. According to your level of comfort, adjust the stretch.

Adapting for Comfort:

1. Chair Support: If your hips are sensitive, place cushions or folded blankets under your knees for support.

2. Gentle Forward Lean: Feel free to skip the forward lean if it causes any discomfort in your hips or back.

Integration and Reflection:

Seated Butterfly Stretch is an invitation to honor the fluidity and grace within your body, even while seated. Through this pose, you create a sense of openness and relaxation, allowing your body to unfurl like the delicate wings of a butterfly. Infuse Seated Butterfly Stretch into your chair yoga practice, allowing it to be a gentle reminder that in every moment, you have the opportunity to nurture your flexibility, embrace tranquility, and unfold into a deeper connection with your body's wisdom.

Seated Leg Extension: Promoting Leg Strength and Flexibility

Seated Leg Extension, a versatile exercise, empowers you to engage and stretch your leg muscles while comfortably seated in your chair. This movement offers seniors a way to strengthen their legs, enhance flexibility, and bring awareness to the engagement of their lower body. Let's explore the essence of Seated Leg Extension and uncover the empowering benefits it brings to your chair yoga practice.

Setting the Foundation:

1. Initial Position: Begin by sitting near the edge of your chair, with your spine tall and your feet flat on the ground.

2. Hand Placement: Place your hands on the sides of the chair for support, maintaining a relaxed and upright posture.

Exploring the Exercise:

1. Engage Your Core: Gently activate your core muscles by drawing your navel toward your spine.

2. Lift Your Leg: Extend one leg forward, keeping your foot flexed and your toes pointing toward the ceiling.

3. Knee Softness: To avoid locking your knee, maintain a slight bend in your extended leg.

4. Hold and Release: Hold the leg extension for a few seconds, feeling the engagement in your thigh muscles, and then release.

Benefits Beyond Strength:

1. Leg Strength: Seated Leg Extension targets the quadriceps, helping to build strength in the front of your thighs.

2. Leg Flexibility: The exercise encourages flexibility as you extend your leg, promoting mobility in the hip joint.

3. Mindful Awareness: Engaging and extending your leg promotes mindfulness, bringing attention to the movement and the sensations in your muscles.

Mindful Engagement:

1. Breath Alignment: Inhale as you prepare to extend your leg, and exhale as you hold the leg extension.

2. Muscle Sensation: As you lift and hold your leg, tune into the sensations in your thigh muscles. Notice the engagement and any areas of tension.

Comfort and Adaptations:

1. Chair Support: If you have limited mobility, use your hands to gently hold your knee as you extend your leg.

2. Gentle Movement: If extending your leg fully is challenging, focus on a gentle and comfortable extension that feels manageable for your body.

Integration and Reflection:

Seated Leg Extension is a testament to the power of simple movements that nurture strength and flexibility. Through this exercise, you honor the vitality and potential of your legs, embracing the balance between strength and subtlety. Infuse Seated Leg Extension into your chair yoga practice, allowing it to empower your lower body, foster mindfulness, and serve as a gentle reminder that within every movement, you have the opportunity to connect with your body's resilience and wisdom.

Seated Hamstring Stretch: Cultivating Leg Flexibility and Comfort

The Seated Hamstring Stretch, a gentle and effective exercise, allows you to stretch and lengthen the muscles of your hamstrings while comfortably seated in your chair. This movement offers seniors a way to promote flexibility in the back of their legs, enhance circulation, and experience a soothing sense of release. Let's explore the essence of Seated Hamstring Stretch and uncover the nurturing benefits it brings to your chair yoga practice.

Creating a Comfortable Base:

1. Initial Position: Sit on the edge of your chair, with your spine tall and your feet flat on the ground.

2. Leg Position: Extend one leg straight in front of you, keeping your foot flexed and your toes pointing toward the ceiling.

3. Hand Placement: Rest your hands on your thighs or on the sides of the chair for support.

Exploring the Stretch:

1. Engage Your Core: Gently activate your core muscles by drawing your navel toward your spine.

2. Hinge Forward: While maintaining a straight spine, lean slightly forward from your hips toward the extended leg.

3. Lengthen Your Spine: Imagine your spine lengthening as you hinge forward, creating space between each vertebra.

4. Feel the Stretch: You'll begin to feel a gentle stretch along the back of the extended leg, targeting the hamstrings.

Benefits Beyond Flexibility:

1. Hamstring Flexibility: Seated Hamstring Stretch encourages gentle lengthening of the hamstring muscles, promoting flexibility.

2. Lower Back Release: As you hinge forward, you may experience a sense of release and relaxation in the lower back.

3. Circulation Enhancement: The movement can help increase blood flow to the legs and alleviate stiffness.

4. Mindful Connection: Seated Hamstring Stretch invites you to connect with the sensations in your body and practice mindful movement.

Mindful Stretching:

1. Breath Alignment: Inhale deeply as you prepare to hinge forward, and exhale as you find a comfortable stretch.

2. Sensory Awareness: As you lean forward, notice the sensations in your hamstring muscles. Pay attention to any areas of tightness or release.

Comfort and Adaptations:

1. Chair Support: If you have limited flexibility, use your hands to gently support your back and help you maintain an upright spine.

2. Gentle Lean: Focus on a gentle and comfortable forward lean that feels appropriate for your body's flexibility.

Integration and Reflection:

Seated Hamstring Stretch is an opportunity to honor the flexibility and resilience of your legs while respecting the uniqueness of your body. Through this stretch, you create a moment of self-care and a gentle connection with the sensations within your muscles. Infuse Seated Hamstring Stretch into your chair yoga practice, allowing it to be a mindful journey of exploration, a pathway to greater flexibility, and a reminder that within every stretch, you have the chance to embrace your body's wisdom and the beauty of slow, intentional movement.

Seated Neck Stretch: Embracing Relaxation and Release

The Seated Neck Stretch offers a serene and calming way to release tension and invite relaxation into your chair yoga practice. This gentle stretch allows seniors to nurture their neck muscles, promote flexibility, and experience a sense of peacefulness. Let's explore the essence of the Seated Neck

Stretch and discover the soothing benefits it brings to your practice.

Creating a Comfortable Seat:

1. Initial Position: Sit comfortably on the edge of your chair, with your spine tall and your feet grounded.

2. Hand Placement: Place your hands on your thighs, allowing them to rest gently.

Exploring the Stretch:

1. Mindful Posture: Ensure your spine is aligned and your shoulders are relaxed.

2. Tilt Your Ear: Gently tilt your head to one side, bringing your ear toward your shoulder.

3. Stay Relaxed: Allow the weight of your head to create a gentle stretch along the side of your neck.

4. Mindful Breathe: Take slow, deep breaths as you hold the stretch, allowing the breath to enhance the sensation of relaxation.

Benefits Beyond Relaxation:

1. Tension Release: Seated Neck Stretch targets the neck muscles, which often hold tension due to everyday activities.

2. Neck Flexibility: The stretch promotes flexibility in the neck, enhancing your range of motion.

3. Stress Relief: As you focus on the stretch and the breath, you may experience a calming effect on the nervous system.

4. Mind-Body Connection: Seated Neck Stretch offers an opportunity to cultivate mindfulness and presence as you connect with the sensations in your neck.

Mindful Stretching:

1. Breath Awareness: Inhale deeply as you prepare to tilt your head, and exhale as you gently guide your ear toward your shoulder.

2. Sensory Connection: As you hold the stretch, pay attention to the sensations in your neck. Any regions of tension or relaxation should be noted.

Comfort and Adaptations:

1. Gentle Movement: Move slowly and gently, ensuring you don't strain your neck muscles.

2. Hold and Breathe: Hold the stretch for a few breaths on each side, allowing time for relaxation.

Integration and Reflection:

Seated Neck Stretch offers you the gift of a tranquil moment: a moment to release and soften the often-overworked muscles of your neck. Through this stretch, you honor your body's capacity to find calm within movement and stillness alike. Infuse Seated Neck Stretch into your chair yoga practice, allowing it to be a gentle reminder that within every stretch, you can discover a sanctuary of peace, a pathway to relaxation, and a connection with the wisdom that resides within your body.

Seated Child's Pose: Embracing Rest and Inner Stillness

Seated Child's Pose, a comforting and introspective posture, offers a way to find rest and surrender within your chair yoga practice. This gentle stretch allows seniors to nurture a sense of inner calm, promote relaxation, and experience a gentle release in their back and shoulders. Let's delve into the essence of Seated Child's Pose and uncover the nourishing benefits it brings to your practice.

Creating a Serene Foundation:

1. Initial Position: Sit comfortably on your chair, with your spine tall and your feet flat on the ground.

2. Hand Placement: Rest your hands on your lap or thighs, palms facing down.

Exploring the Posture:

1. Mindful Posture: Sit tall and align your spine while maintaining a sense of relaxation.

2. Forward Fold: Gently lean forward from your hips, allowing your chest to rest on your thighs.

3. Arm Position: Extend your arms forward along the sides of your legs, creating a sense of length in your spine.

4. Relaxation: Allow your forehead to rest on your legs or on a cushion placed on your lap.

Benefits Beyond Rest:

1. Relaxation and Surrender: Seated Child's Pose encourages a sense of surrender and relaxation, fostering inner tranquility.

2. Shoulder and Back Release: The gentle forward fold can create a soothing stretch in the shoulders, upper back, and spine.

3. Breath Awareness: As you rest in the pose, observe the rhythm of your breath, inviting a calm and meditative state.

4. Mindful Pause: Seated Child's Pose offers an opportunity to pause, turn inward, and connect with the present moment.

Mindful Presence:

1. Breath Connection: Inhale deeply as you sit tall, and exhale as you fold forward. Allow your breath to guide you into relaxation.

2. Sensory Reflection: As you hold the posture, tune into the sensations of your breath, the gentle stretch, and the support of the chair beneath you.

Comfort and Adaptations:

1. Chair Support: If leaning forward is uncomfortable, rest your forearms on your thighs, and focus on a gentle forward tilt.

2. Cushion Comfort: If your forehead doesn't comfortably reach your legs, place a cushion or folded blanket on your lap for support.

Integration and Reflection:

Seated Child's Pose invites you to find solace and rejuvenation within the simplicity of stillness and breath. Through this pose, you honor your body's need for rest and restoration, embracing the nourishing embrace of the present moment. Infuse Seated Child's Pose into your chair yoga practice, allowing it to be a gentle sanctuary where you can soften, connect with the essence of tranquility, and discover the profound beauty of inner stillness.

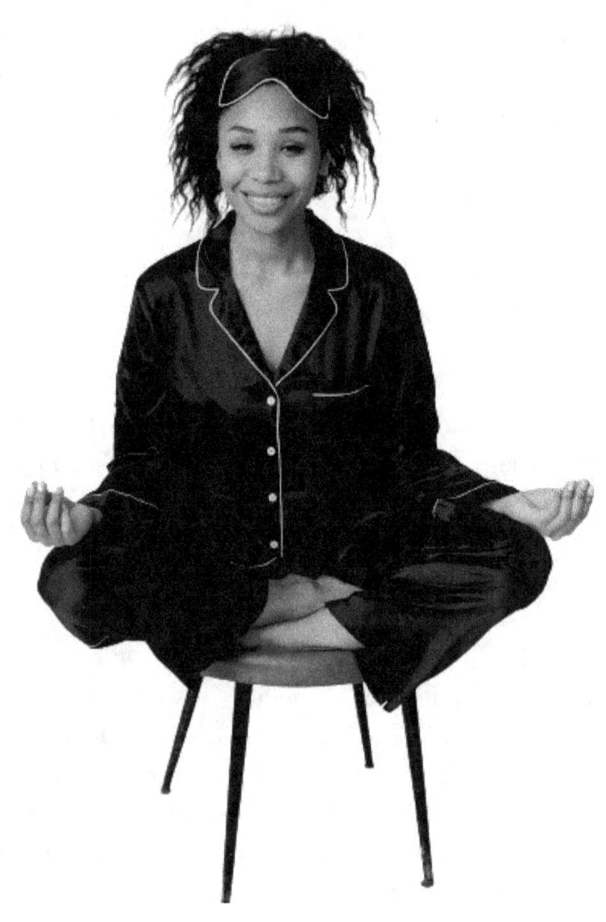

Seated Savasana: Embracing Deep Relaxation and Renewal

Seated Savasana, a soothing and contemplative pose, offers a way to experience deep relaxation and rejuvenation within your chair yoga practice. This restful posture allows seniors to unwind, let go of tension, and cultivate a sense of inner stillness and renewal. Let's explore the essence of Seated Savasana and discover the rejuvenating benefits it brings to your practice.

Creating a Restful Seat:

1. Initial Position: Sit comfortably on your chair, with your spine tall and your feet flat on the ground.

2. Hand Placement: Rest your hands on your lap or thighs, palms facing up or down, as feels comfortable.

Exploring the Pose:

1. Mindful Posture: Find a comfortable and supported seat, allowing your body to relax into the chair.

2. Close Your Eyes: Gently close your eyes to turn your focus inward and minimize distractions.

3. Relax and Let Go: Allow your body to relax, releasing any tension you might be holding.

4. Breath Awareness: Bring your attention to your breath, observing its natural rhythm without trying to change it.

Benefits Beyond Relaxation:

1. Deep Relaxation: Seated Savasana encourages profound relaxation, helping to calm the nervous system and reduce stress.

2. Mindful Presence: The pose invites you to cultivate mindfulness by focusing on your breath and observing the sensations within your body.

3. Renewal and Recharge: By allowing yourself this moment of rest, you create an opportunity for rejuvenation and renewed energy.

4. Inner Stillness: Seated Savasana offers a space for inner quietude, allowing you to connect with a sense of tranquility within.

Mindful Reflection:

1. Breath Connection: Softly inhale and exhale, allowing your breath to be your guide as you settle into the pose.

2. Sensory Awareness: As you rest in Seated Savasana, gently observe any sensations within your body, and let them come and go without attachment.

Comfort and Adaptations:

1. Chair Support: If sitting upright is challenging, you can rest your back against the backrest of the chair for added support.

2. Cushion Comfort: Place a cushion or folded blanket on your lap for extra comfort and warmth.

Integration and Reflection:

Seated Savasana is a sanctuary of stillness and reflection, a place where you can allow the layers of busyness to gently fall away, revealing the quietude that resides within. Through this pose, you honor your body's need for rest and invite the soothing embrace of tranquility. Infuse Seated Savasana into your chair yoga practice, allowing it to be a moment of self-care, a pause to connect with your breath, and an opportunity to renew your spirit, one conscious breath at a time.

Deep Breathing: Cultivating Calmness and Inner Balance

Deep breathing, also known as diaphragmatic or abdominal breathing, is a simple yet powerful practice that can bring a sense of calmness and balance to your body and mind. This practice involves intentionally taking slow, deep breaths to activate the diaphragm and promote relaxation. Let's explore the essence of deep breathing and uncover the serene benefits it brings to your chair yoga practice.

Preparing for Deep Breathing:

1. Initial Position: Sit comfortably on your chair, with your spine tall and your feet grounded.

2. Hand Placement: Place your hands on your lap or thighs, palms facing up or down.

Exploring the Practice:

1. Mindful Posture: Find a comfortable and supported seat, allowing your body to relax.

2. Close Your Eyes: Gently close your eyes to minimize external distractions and turn your focus inward.

3. Inhale Deeply: Inhale slowly and deeply through your nose, allowing your breath to fill your abdomen.

4. Expand Your Belly: As you inhale, feel your abdomen gently rise, expanding as your diaphragm moves downward.

5. Exhale Completely: Exhale slowly and fully through your nose or mouth, emptying your lungs completely.

6. Release Your Breath: As you exhale, feel your abdomen gently fall, releasing any residual tension.

Benefits Beyond Relaxation:

1. Stress Reduction: Deep breathing activates the body's relaxation response, helping to reduce stress and anxiety.

2. Calming the Mind: The practice encourages a calm and centered state of mind, promoting mental clarity.

3. Oxygenation: Deep breaths bring more oxygen into the body, promoting better oxygen exchange and overall vitality.

4. Mind-Body Connection: Deep breathing invites you to connect with the present moment, fostering mindfulness.

Mindful Breathing:

1. Breath Awareness: Pay attention to the sensation of the breath as it moves in and out of your body. Observe the rise and fall of your abdomen.

2. Rhythm of Breath: Allow your breath to flow naturally, without force. Find a rhythm that feels comfortable and soothing.

Comfort and Adaptations:

1. Chair Support: If sitting upright is challenging, use the backrest of the chair to support your posture.

2. Hand Placement: Rest your hands on your abdomen to feel the rise and fall of your breath more clearly.

Integration and Reflection:

Deep breathing is a gift you can offer yourself at any moment a way to return to your breath and find solace within its rhythmic flow. Through this practice, you embrace the simplicity and depth of each inhalation and exhalation. Infuse deep breathing into your chair yoga practice, allowing it to be a thread of serenity woven into each movement, a reminder to come back to the present moment, and a bridge to the stillness that resides within you.

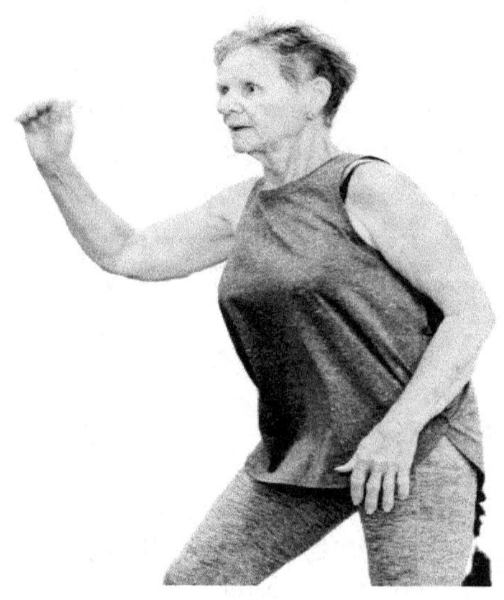

Conclusion

As we conclude this journey through the world of chair yoga for seniors, we reflect on the tapestry of balance, mindfulness, and well-being that we've woven together. Chair yoga isn't just about physical movement; it's a path to cultivating harmony between body, mind, and spirit. Throughout these pages, we've explored the gentle embrace of poses that honor your unique needs and celebrate the vitality that resides within you.

From the captivating benefits of chair yoga that extend far beyond the physical, to the safety precautions and guidelines that ensure your practice is your sanctuary, this book has been your guide to a holistic approach to wellness. We've learned that even the simple act of breathing and the mindful stretch of a muscle can be a gateway to serenity. With each page turned, you've embarked on a journey of self-care, one that encourages you to listen to your body's wisdom and honor your journey.

Choosing the right chair, embracing comfortable clothing and a nurturing environment, and practicing foundational poses have all been stepping stones on your path to wellness. From Seated Mountain Pose to Seated Savasana, you've explored a spectrum of movements that honor your body's range and promote strength, flexibility, and balance.

As you journey through this book, may you have found not only physical benefits but also a deeper connection with your inner self. Chair yoga isn't just about poses; it's about finding a space within yourself where you can breathe, move, and be present. In each moment of practice, you've embraced the beauty of mindful movement, connecting with the essence of tranquility.

Remember, the wisdom of chair yoga extends beyond the pages of this book. Carry the spirit of balance, mindfulness, and well-being with you, allowing it to permeate every facet of your life. Whether you find yourself in the comfort of your home, in a serene garden, or amidst the bustling world, the practice of chair yoga is your sanctuary, a space where you can find respite, renewal, and a deeper connection with your own vitality.

As you continue on your journey, may the lessons learned from chair yoga guide you to a place of wellness, resilience, and joy. Embrace each breath, each stretch, and each moment as an opportunity to honor yourself and the vibrant spirit that you are. From the seated poses to the expansive universe within, may your journey be one of self-discovery, nurturing, and a celebration of life's beautiful tapestry.

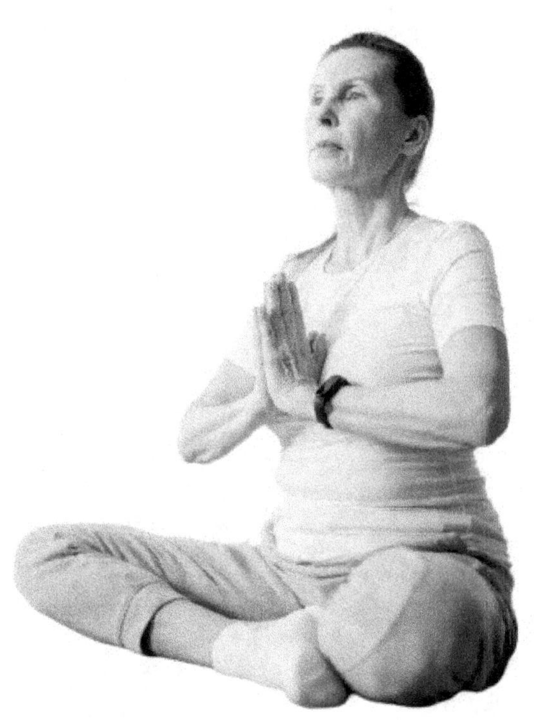